The Complete Lean and Green Diet Plan

I0145893

50 step-by-step and affordable recipes for your Lean and Green diet, delicious, easy to prepare to burn fat fast

Josephine Reed

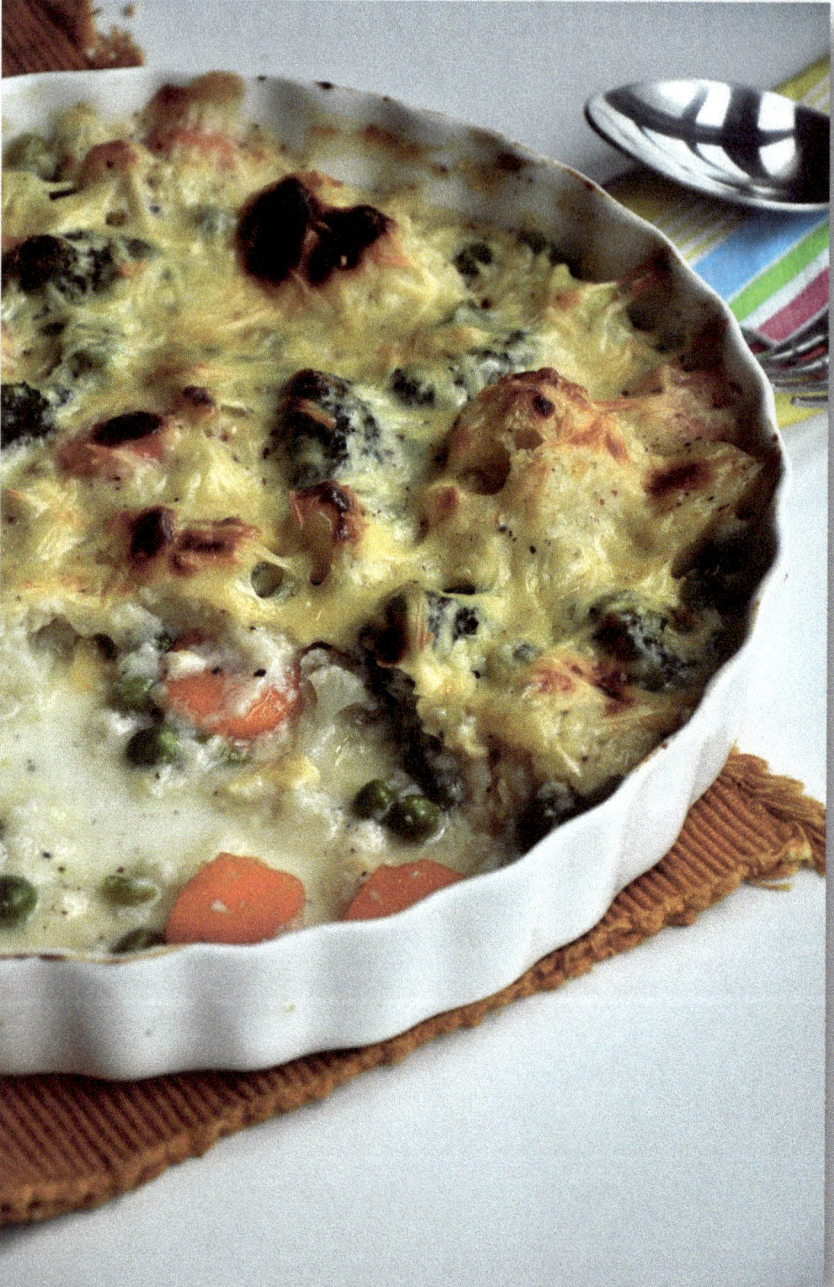

Please consult a licensed professional before attempting any techniques outlined in this book.

By reading this document, the reader agrees that under no circumstances is the author responsible for any losses, direct or indirect, which are incurred as a result of the use of information contained within this document, including, but not limited to, — errors, omissions, or inaccuracies.

Table of contents

Tofu Scramble

Time: 17 minutes

Serve: 2

Ingredients:

- 1/2 block firm tofu, crumbled
- 1 cup spinach
- 1/4 cup zucchini, chopped
- 1 tbsp olive oil
- 1 tomato, chopped
- 1/4 tsp ground cumin
- 1 tbsp turmeric
- 1 tbsp coriander, chopped
- 1 tbsp chives, chopped
- Pepper and Salt

Instructions:

1.Heat the oil in a pan.

2.Add tomato, zucchini, and spinach and sauté for 2 minutes.

3.Add tofu, turmeric, cumin, pepper, and salt, and sauté for 5 minutes.

4.Garnish with chives and coriander.

Nutrition: Calories 102 Fat 8 g Carbs 5 g Sugar 2 g Protein 3 g
Cholesterol 0 mg

Shrimp & Zucchini

Time: 30 minutes

Serve: 4

Ingredients:

- 1 lb shrimp, peeled and deveined
- 1 zucchini, chopped
- 1 summer squash, chopped
- 2 tbsp olive oil
- 1/2 small onion, chopped
- 1/2 tsp paprika
- 1/2 tsp garlic powder
- 1/2 tsp onion powder
- Pepper and Salt

Instructions:

1.In a bowl, mix paprika, garlic powder, onion powder, pepper, and salt. Add shrimp and toss well.

2.Heat 1 normal spoon of oil in a pan over medium heat,

3.Add shrimp and cook for 2 minutes on each side or until shrimp turns pink.

4.Transfer shrimp on a plate.

5.Add remaining oil to a pan.

6.Add onion, summer squash, and zucchini, and cook for 6-8 minutes or until vegetables are softened.

7. Place the shrimp-back in the pan and cook for 1 minute.

Nutrition: Calories 215 Fat 9 g Carbs 6 g Sugar 2 g Protein 27 g Cholesterol 239 mg

Baked Dijon Salmon

Time: 30 minutes

Serve: 5

Ingredients:

- 1 1/2 lbs salmon
- 1/4 cup Dijon mustard
- 1/4 cup fresh parsley, chopped
- 1 tbsp garlic, chopped
- 1 tbsp olive oil
- 1 tbsp fresh lemon juice
- Pepper and Salt

Instructions:

1.Preheat the oven to 385 F. Line baking sheet with parchment paper.

2.Arrange salmon fillets on a prepared baking sheet.

3.In a small bowl, mix garlic, oil, lemon juice, Dijon mustard, parsley, pepper, and salt.

4.Brush salmon top with garlic mixture.

5.Bake for 18-20 minutes.

Nutrition: Calories 217 Fat 11 g Carbs 2 g Sugar 0.2 g Protein 27 g Cholesterol 60 mg

Cauliflower Spinach Rice

Time: 15 minutes

Serve: 4

Ingredients:

- 5 oz baby spinach
- 4 cups cauliflower rice
- 1 tsp garlic, minced
- 3 tbsp olive oil
- 1 fresh lime juice
- 1/4 cup vegetable broth
- 1/4 tsp chili powder
- Pepper and Salt

Instructions:

1.Heat the olive oil in a pan.

2.Add garlic and sauté for 30 seconds. Add cauliflower rice, chili powder, pepper, and salt and cook for 2 minutes.

3.Add broth and lime juice and stir well.

4.Add spinach and stir until spinach is wilted.

Nutrition: Calories 147 Fat 11 g Carbs 9 g Sugar 4 g Protein 5 g Cholesterol 23 mg

Cauliflower Broccoli Mash

Time: 22 minutes

Serve: 3

Ingredients:

- 1 lb cauliflower, cut into florets
- 2 cups broccoli, chopped
- 1 tsp garlic, minced
- 1 tsp dried rosemary
- 1/4 cup olive oil
- Salt

Instructions:

1.Add broccoli and cauliflower into the instant pot.

2.Pour enough water into the instant pot to cover broccoli and cauliflower.

3.Seal pot and cook on high-pressure for 12 minutes.

4.Once done, allow to release pressure naturally. Remove lid.

5.Drain broccoli and cauliflower and clean the instant pot.

6.Add oil into the instant pot and set the pot on sauté mode.

7.Add broccoli, cauliflower, rosemary, garlic, and salt, and cook for 10 minutes.

8.Mash the broccoli and cauliflower mixture using a masher until smooth.

Nutrition: Calories 205 Fat 17 g Carbs 12 g Sugar 5 g Protein 5 g Cholesterol 0 mg

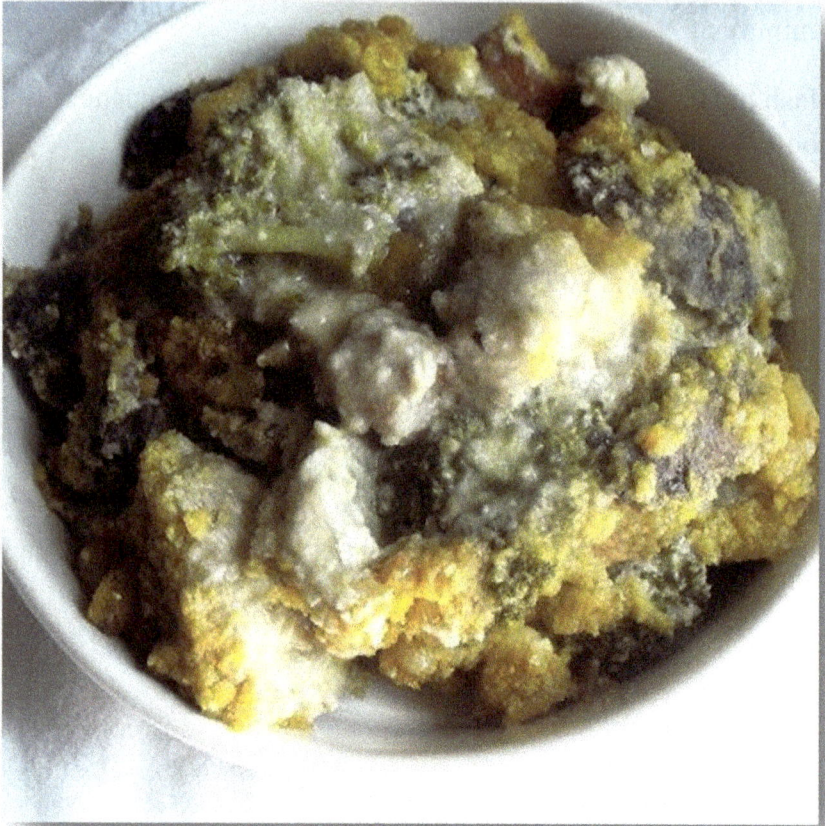

Italian Chicken Soup

Time: 35 minutes

Serve: 6

Ingredients:

- 1 lb chicken breasts, boneless and cut into chunks
- 1 1/2 cups salsa
- 1 tsp Italian seasoning
- 2 tbsp fresh parsley, chopped
- 3 cups chicken stock
- 8 oz cream cheese
- Pepper and Salt

Instructions:

1.Add all ingredients except cream cheese and parsley into the instant pot and stir well.

2.Seal pot and cook on high-pressure for 25 minutes.

3.Release pressure using quick release. Remove lid.

4.Remove chicken from pot and shred using a fork.

5.Return shredded chicken to the instant pot.

6.Add cream cheese and stir well and cook on sauté mode until cheese is melted.

Nutrition: Calories 300 Fat 19 g Carbs 5 g Sugar 2 g Protein 26 g Cholesterol 109 mg

Tasty Tomatoes Soup

Time: 15 minutes

Serve: 2

Ingredients:

- 14 oz can fire-roasted tomatoes
- 1/2 tsp dried basil
- 1/2 cup heavy cream
- 1/2 cup parmesan cheese, grated
- 1 cup cheddar cheese, grated
- 1 1/2 cups vegetable stock
- 1/4 cup zucchini, grated
- 1/2 tsp dried oregano
- Pepper and Salt

Instructions:

1.Add tomatoes, stock, zucchini, oregano, basil, pepper, and salt into the instant pot and stir well.

2.Seal pot and cook on high-pressure for 5 minutes.

3.Release pressure using quick release. Remove lid.

4.Set pot on sauté mode. Add heavy cream, parmesan cheese, and cheddar cheese and stir well and cook until cheese is melted.

Nutrition: Calories 460 Fat 35 g Carbs 13 g Sugar 6 g Protein 24 g Cholesterol 117 mg

Cauliflower Spinach Soup

Time: 20 minutes

Serve: 2

Ingredients:

- 3 cups spinach, chopped
- 1 cup cauliflower, chopped
- 2 tbsp olive oil
- 3 cups vegetable broth
- 1/2 cup heavy cream
- 1 tsp garlic powder
- Pepper
- Salt

Instructions:

1.Add all ingredients except cream into the instant pot and stir well.

2.Seal pot and cook on high-pressure for 11 minutes.

3.Release pressure using quick release. Remove lid.

4.Stir in cream and blend soup using a blender until smooth.

Nutrition: Calories 310 Fat 27 g Carbs 7 g Sugar 3 g Protein 10 g Cholesterol 41 mg

Delicious Chicken Salad

Time: 15 minutes

Serve: 4

Ingredients:

- 1 1/2 cups chicken breast, skinless, boneless, and cooked
- 2 tbsp onion, diced
- 1/4 cup olives, diced
- 1/4 cup roasted red peppers, diced
- 1/4 cup cucumbers, diced
- 1/4 cup celery, diced
- 1/4 cup feta cheese, crumbled
- 1/2 tsp onion powder
- 1/2 tbsp fresh lemon juice
- 1 tbsp fresh parsley, chopped
- 1 tbsp fresh dill, chopped
- 2 1/2 tbsp mayonnaise
- 1/4 cup Greek yogurt
- 1/4 tsp pepper
- 1/2 tsp salt

Instructions:

1.In a bowl, mix yogurt, onion powder, lemon juice, parsley, dill, mayonnaise, pepper, and salt.

2.Add chicken, onion, olives, red peppers, cucumbers, and feta cheese and stir well.

Nutrition: Calories 172 Fat 7.9 g Carbs 6.7 g Sugar 3.1 g Protein 18.1 g Cholesterol 52 mg

Baked Pesto Salmon

Time: 30 minutes

Serve: 5

Ingredients:

- 1 3/4 lbs salmon fillet
- 1/3 cup basil pesto
- 1/4 cup sun-dried tomatoes, drained
- 1/4 cup olives, pitted and chopped
- 1 tbsp fresh dill, chopped
- 1/4 cup capers
- 1/3 cup artichoke hearts
- 1 tsp paprika
- 1/4 tsp salt

Instructions:

1.Preheat the oven to 410 F. Cover the pan with parchment paper.

2.Arrange salmon fillet on a prepared baking sheet and season with paprika and salt.

3.Add remaining ingredients on top of salmon and spread evenly.

4.Bake for 20 minutes.

Nutrition: Calories 228 Fat 10.7 g Carbs 2.7 g Sugar 0.3 g Protein 31.6 g Cholesterol 70 mg

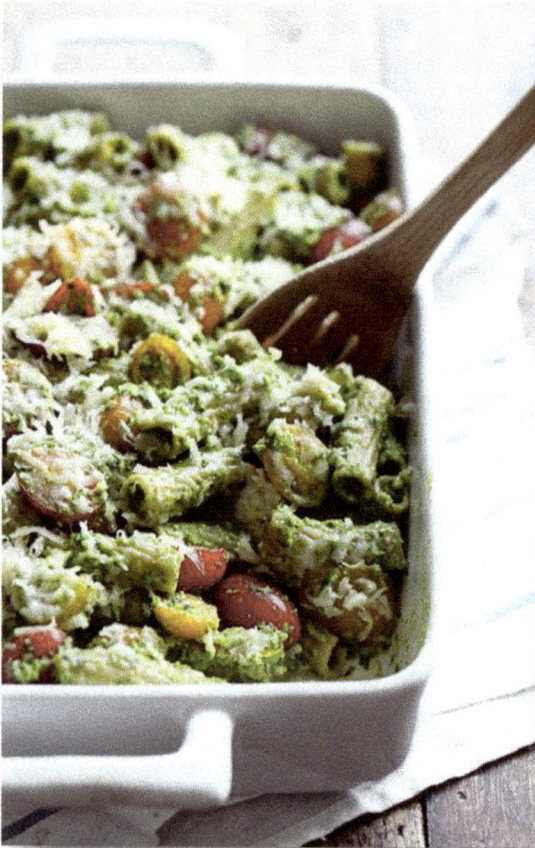

Easy Shrimp Salad

Time: 15 minutes

Serve: 6

Ingredients:

- 2 lbs shrimp, cooked
- 1/4 cup onion, minced
- 1/4 cup fresh dill, chopped
- 1/3 cup fresh chives, chopped
- 1/2 cup fresh celery, chopped
- 1/4 tsp cayenne pepper
- 1 tbsp fresh lemon juice
- 1 tbsp olive oil
- 1/4 cup mayonnaise
- 1/4 tsp pepper
- 1/4 tsp salt

Instructions:

1.In a big-bowl, add all ingredients except shrimp and mix well.

2.Add shrimp and toss well.

Nutrition: Calories 248 Fat 8.3 g Carbs 6.7 g Sugar 1.1 g Protein 35.2 g Cholesterol 321 mg

Simple Haddock Salad

Time: 15 minutes

Serve: 6

Ingredients:

- 1 lb haddock, cooked
- 1 tbsp green onion, chopped
- 1 tbsp olive oil
- 1 tsp garlic, minced
- Pepper and Salt

Instructions:

1. Cut cooked haddock into bite-size pieces and place on a plate.

2. Season with oil, pepper, and salt

3. Sprinkle garlic and green onion over haddock.

Nutrition: Calories 106 Fat 3 g Carbs 0.2 g Sugar 0 g Protein 18.4 g Cholesterol 56 mg

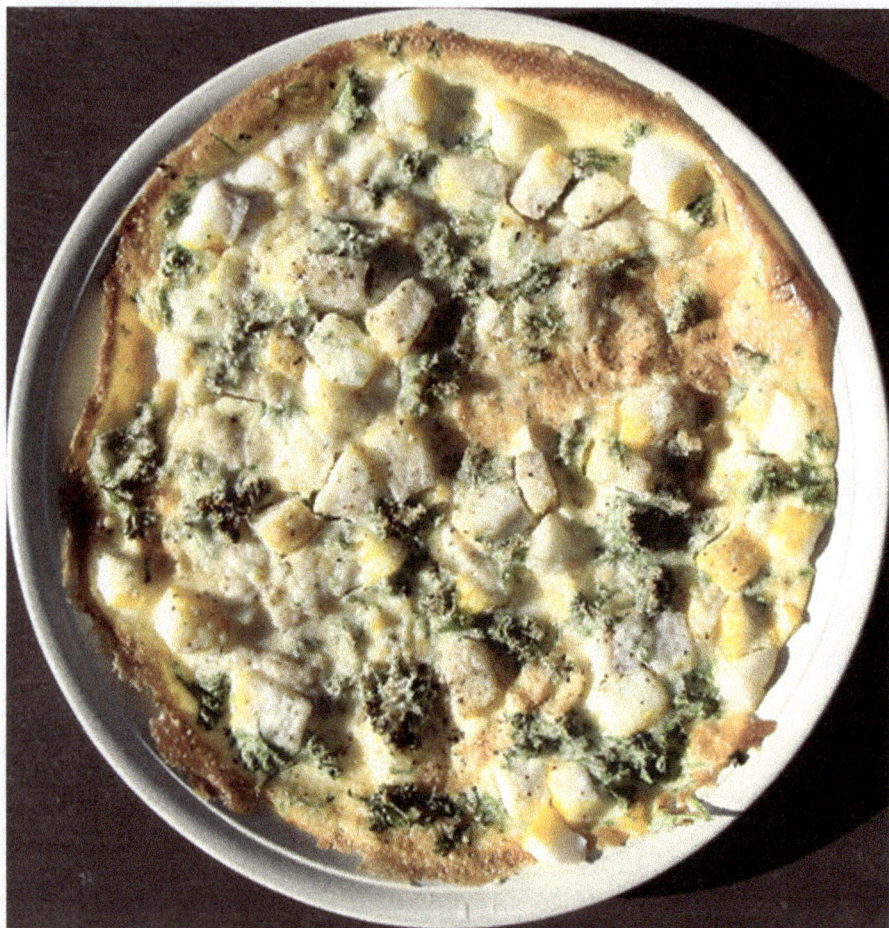

Baked White Fish Fillet

Time: 40 minutes

Serve: 1

Ingredients:

- 8 oz frozen white fish fillet
- 1 tbsp roasted red bell pepper, diced
- 1/2 tsp Italian seasoning
- 1 tbsp fresh parsley, chopped
- 1 1/2 tbsp olive oil
- 1 tbsp lemon juice

Instructions:

1.Preheat the oven to 410 F. Line baking sheet with foil.

2.Place a fish fillet on a baking sheet.

3.Drizzle oil and lemon juice over fish. Season with Italian seasoning.

4.Top with roasted bell pepper and parsley and bake for 30 minutes.

Nutrition: Calories 383 Fat 22.5 g Carbs 0.8 g Sugar 0.6 g Protein 46.5 g Cholesterol 2 mg

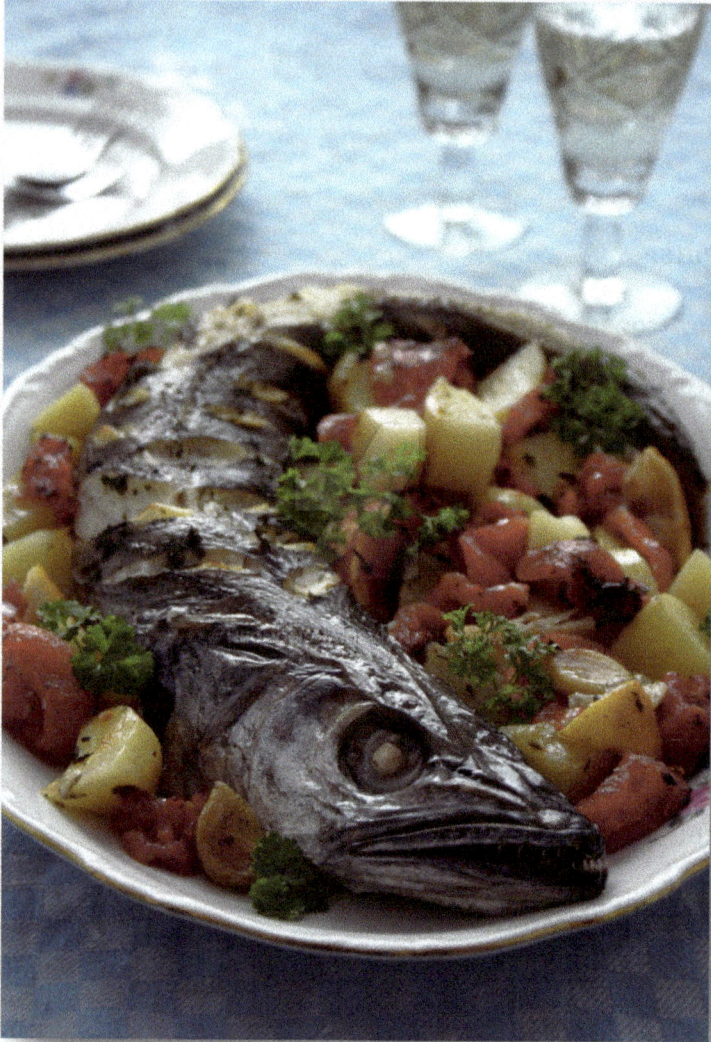

Air Fry Salmon

Time: 25 minutes

Serve: 4

Ingredients:

- 1 lbs salmon, cut into 4 pieces
- 1 tbsp olive oil
- 1/2 tbsp dried rosemary
- 1/4 tsp dried basil
- 1 tbsp dried chives
- Pepper and Salt

Instructions:

1.Place salmon-pieces skin side down into the air fryer basket.

2.In a small bowl, mix olive oil, basil, chives, and rosemary.

3.Brush salmon with oil mixture and air fry at 400 F for 15 minutes.

Nutrition: Calories 182 Fat 10.6 g Carbs 0.3 g Sugar 0 g Protein 22 g Cholesterol 50 mg

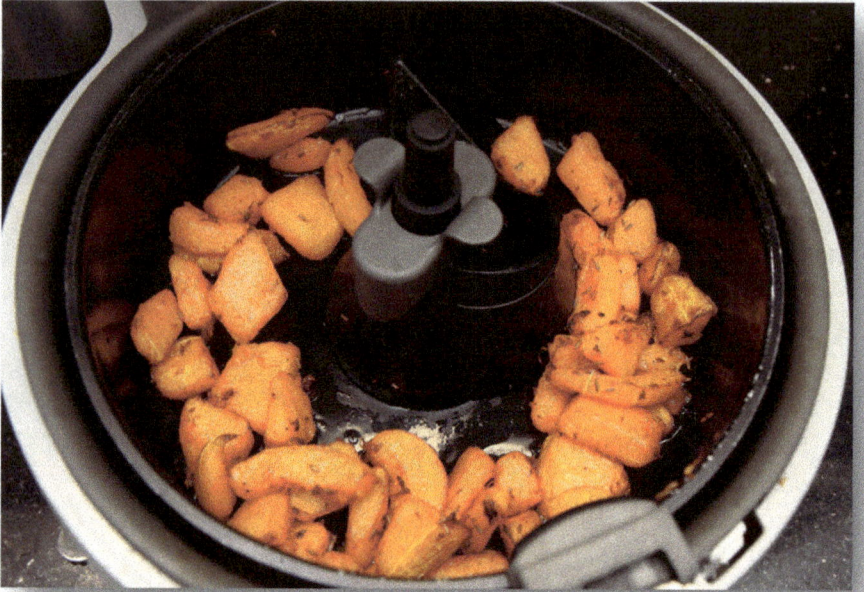

Baked Salmon Patties

Time: 30 minutes

Serve: 4

Ingredients:

- 2 eggs, lightly beaten
- 14 oz can salmon, drained and flaked with a fork
- 1 tbsp garlic, minced
- 1/4 cup almond flour
- 1/2 cup fresh parsley, chopped
- 1 tsp Dijon mustard
- 1/4 tsp pepper
- 1/2 tsp kosher salt

Instructions:

1. Preheat a 410 F microwave. Line a baking sheet and set it aside with parchment paper.

2. Add all ingredients into the bowl and mix until well combined.

3. Make small patties from the mixture and place on a prepared baking sheet.

4. Bake patties for 10 minutes.

5.Turn patties and bake for 10 minutes more.

Nutrition: Calories 216 Fat 11.8 g Carbs 3 g Sugar 0.5 g Protein 24.3 g Cholesterol 136 mg

Peanut Butter Banana Sandwich

Prep Time: 2 minutes

Cook Time: 6 minutes

Serve: 1

Ingredients:

- 1 banana
- 1 tbsp. olive oil (or coconut oil)
- ½ tbsp. cinnamon
- 1 tbsp. peanut butter
- slices bread

Instructions:

1. On both slices of toast, smear the peanut butter.

2. Slice the banana into thin slices about 8 mm thick and spread them on just ONE toast slice.

3. Over them, add cinnamon.

4. Place all slices on each other's top.

5. For 2-3 minutes, apply oil to the pan and cook both faces until crispy and brown and yummy and delicious, and boom! Now, back to bed.

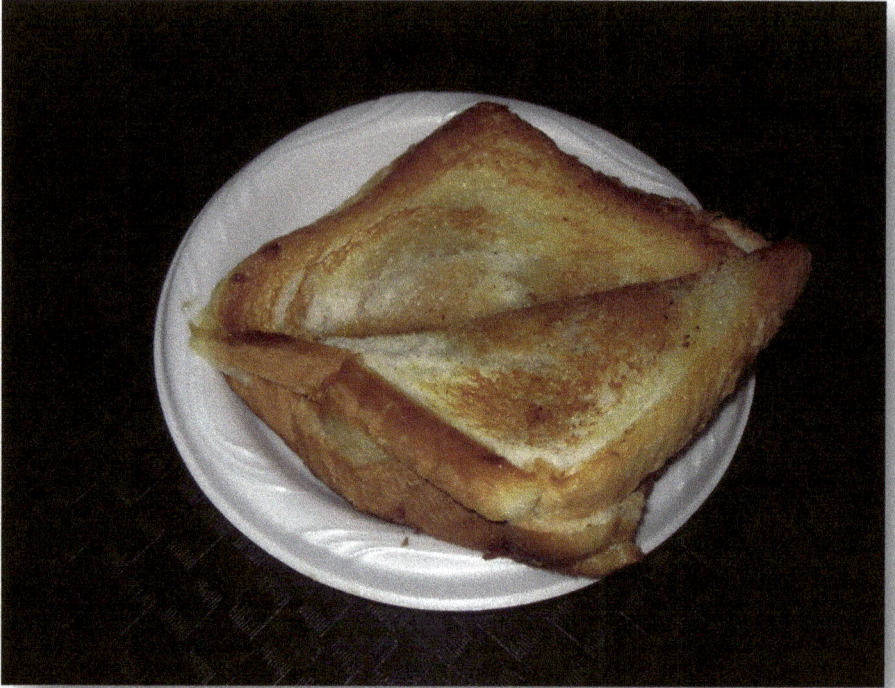

Tuna Pate

Prep Time: 15 min

Cook Time: 45 min

Serve: 6

Ingredients:

- 1/4 teaspoon pepper
- 1/4 teaspoon salt
- Grated rind of half an orange
- 2 tablespoons fresh parsley
- 1 can (6 ounces) tuna, drained
- 1 package (8 ounces) cream cheese, softened
- 1 can (4 ounces) mushrooms, drained
- 1/2 teaspoon orange extract
- 1 tablespoon Splendor
- 1/2 medium onion, chopped
- 2 cloves garlic, crushed
- 2 tablespoons butter

Instruction:

1. Melt the butter and stir-fry the onion and garlic, and mushrooms in a thin, heavy skillet over low heat until the onion is floppy. Connect the orange and Splendor extract and blend well.

2. With the S blade in, put the tuna, cream cheese, orange rind, parsley, salt, and pepper in a food mixer. Pulse for mixing. Add the sautéed mixture, and pulse until well combined and smooth.

3. Cool and spoon into a mixing dish. Serve with (for carb-eaters) pepper strips, cucumber rounds, celery sticks, and crackers.

Nutrition: 3 g. carb. | 1 g. fib. for a total of 2 g. of usable carbs and 11 grams of protein.

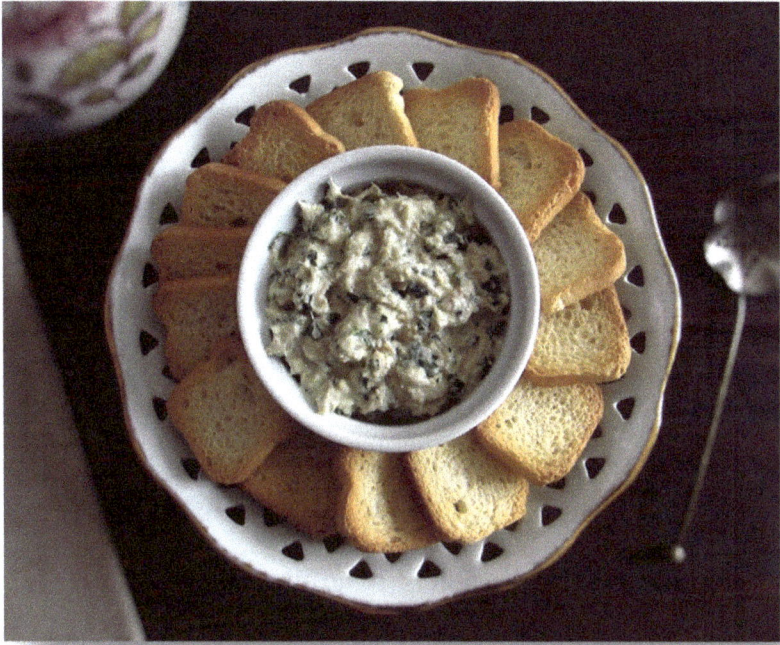

Arugula Lentil Salad

Prep Time: 5 minutes

Cook Time: 7 minutes

Serve: 2

Ingredients:

- 1-2 tbsp. balsamic vinegar
- ¾ cups cashews (¾ cups = 100 g)
- 1 handful arugula/rocket (1 handful = 100 g)
- 1 cup brown lentils, cooked (1 cup = 1 / 15oz. / 400 g)
- slices bread (whole wheat)
- 5-6 sun-dried tomatoes in oil
- 1 chili / jalapeño
- tbsp. olive oil
- 1 onion
- salt and pepper to taste
- Optional
- 1 tbsp. honey
- 1 small handful of raisins

Instructions:

1. To optimize the scent, toast the cashews in a pan over low heat for about three to four minutes. Then dump them into a pot of salad.

2.Dice and fry the onion in one-third of the olive oil over low heat for around 3 minutes.

3.In the meantime, cut your chili / jalapeño and dried tomatoes. In the grill, add them and fry for the next 1-2 minutes.

4.Slice the bread into large croutons.

5.Shift the mixture of onions into a large container. Now add the remaaining oil to the pan and cook the sliced bread until it's crispy with salt and pepper seasoning.

6.Now clean the arugula and put it in the bowl.

7.Bring in the lentils, too, and blend everything over. Using salt, pepper, and balsamic vinegar to season. With the croutons, eat.

Tomato Avocado Toast

Prep Time: 5 min

Cook Time: 5 min

Serve: 1

Ingredients:

- 1 slice bread (ideally whole grain)
- ½ medium avocado (½ avocado = about 50g)
- 1 tbsp. lemon juice
- 1 tbsp. olive oil
- salt and pepper to taste
- cherry tomatoes

Instructions:

1.Split in half your cherry tomatoes.

2.Dump them in a pan and let them cook until tender (about 5 minutes) with olive oil.

3.In the meantime, mash and add some lemon with your avocado. Put it all together now, and season with salt and pepper.

Classic Tofu Salad

Prep Time: 5 minutes

Cook Time: 15 minutes

Serve: 2

Ingredients:

- 1 small tin pineapple (small tin = 8 oz. = 225g = ¼)
- 1 handful spinach
- ½ bunch radishes
- ½ medium cucumber
- 1 cup bean sprouts
- 14 oz. firm tofu (ideally get fresh tofu from the supermarket)

For the dressing

- tbsp. olive oil
- salt and pepper to taste
- 1 small handful of peanuts
- ½ chili pepper (e.g., jalapeño)
- ½ lime (juiced; lemon also works)
- 1 tbsp. sriracha (or equivalent)
- 1 tbsp. maple syrup

Instructions:

1.Squeeze out some of the tofu block's excess moisture, split it (about one square centimeter) into tiny cubes, heat some oil in a pan over low to medium heat, and add it to your tofu. Fry until golden brown for approximately 15 minutes. Challenge for multitasking: make sure that you stir every once in a while (and put some salt). When preparing the rest of the salad, you should do it, get it on!

2.Next step: rinse the vegetables!

3.Chop the radishes.

4.Lengthwise, slice the cucumber in half, scrape the seeds with a big spoon, and cut what's left.

5.Also, cut the pineapple into smaller pieces.

6.Put all together with the bean sprouts and spinach into a dish.

Now to the dressing

1.Put the sugar, the olive oil, the sriracha, the lime juice, the salt, and the pepper together and toss in the salad

2.Get the pieces of tofu and put them in a separate bowl. Mix them to every

3.Serving of salad. (They'll get mushy easily if you put them straight into the salad).

4.Cut the chili and slightly crush or chop the peanuts for garnish as well. When served, dust them over the salad.

Two Ingredient Peanut Butter

Prep Time: 3 min

Cook Time: None

Serve: 8

Ingredients:

- 2 tbsp. olive oil
- 1 tbsp. maple syrup
- 1¼ cup peanuts

Instructions:

1.In a blender/food processor, add chunks of peanuts and oil (add maple syrup if desired).

2.Mix more for smooth texture, less for a crunchy blend.

Avocado Toast with Cottage Cheese

Prep Time: 5 minutes

Cook Time: None

Serve: 1

Ingredients:

- 1 green onion
- 2 tbsp. cottage cheese
- 1 tbsp. lemon
- ½ medium avocado
- 1 slice bread (ideally whole grain)
- salt and pepper to taste

Instructions:

1.Mash the avocado; add the lemon and some salt.

2.On the toast, put a layer of cottage cheese.

3.Garnish with fresh pepper and sliced green onion.

Creamy Corn Soup

Prep Time: 5 minutes

Cook Time: 15 minutes

Serve: 3

Ingredients:

- 1 pinch pepper (preferably freshly ground black pepper)
- 1 pinch salt
- 2 handfuls cilantro/coriander, fresh
- 2 tbsp. olive oil
- 2 cups vegetable broth (2 cups = ½ liter)
- 1 thumb ginger, fresh (or 1 tbsp. ground ginger)
- 2 cloves garlic
- 1 red pepper *
- 2 onion
- cans sweet corn (ca. 14oz. or 350-400g cans)

Optional and highly recommended:

- 1 tbsp. lemon juice (as an extra twist before serving)
- 2 stalks lemongrass (or 1 tbsp. ground lemongrass)

Instructions:

1.Heat the oven to a temperature of 430 ° F/220 ° C.

2.Flush the sweet corn in a different bowl, but save the water from the can!

3.To the baking tray, add 1/3 of the corn (without the water). Sprinkle with salt, pepper, and oil. Put it on for about 10 minutes in the oven. Stir periodically to make sure the maize is not burning.

4.Meanwhile, heat the remaining spoon of oil in a pan over medium heat.

5.Chop and sauté the onion (slowly fry it).

6.Peel the fresh ginger and chop it and transfer it to the onion. (Keep off a moment if dried ginger is used). For a moment, stir.

7.The garlic is sliced and added to the onion. Stir for around 30-60 seconds when the heat is low.

8.Now's the time to apply that to the mix and swirl for around 30-60 seconds if you're using freshly grated ginger (and optional: ground lemongrass).

9.Put the other 2 cans of corn and the liquid you set aside earlier (with the water / moist / broth from the can). The vegetable broth is also added and brought to a boil.

10.Make tiny slits in the lemongrass and apply them to the soup if you're using fresh lemongrass. Or, to slap the lemongrass a few times, use a wooden spoon. Later, as a whole, you can pull them out, so make sure that they remain in one piece.

11.Let the soup-boil on medium heat for around 10 minutes.

12.Regularly check on your oven-roasted corn. Meanwhile, cut the cilantro and slice the red pepper into small bits. If you don't want it hot, you want the red pepper first.

13.When the roasted corn is done (superbly golden, piping hot, popping here and there), put in the red pepper and coriander together to a cup. Just blend it well.

14.Remove the soup from the heat after ten minutes of boiling and mix it (a hand blender is ideal) until it's (kind of) smooth.

15.Serve the soup with the corn-coriander-red pepper mix in a teaspoon (or two!) of it.

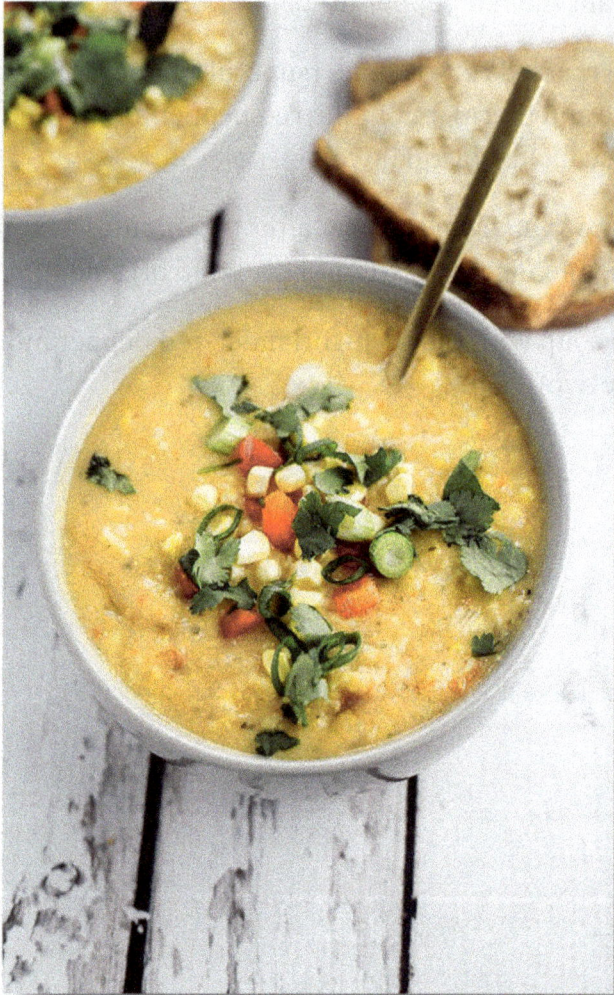

Balsamic Chicken Breast

Prep Time: 10 minutes

Cook Time: 14 minutes

Serve: 4

Ingredients:

- ¼ cup balsamic vinegar
- 2 tablespoons olive oil
- 1½ teaspoons fresh lemon juice
- ½ teaspoon lemon-pepper seasoning
- 4 (6-ounce) boneless, skinless-chicken breast halves, pounded slightly
- 6 cups fresh baby kale

Instructions:

1. In a glass baking dish, place the vinegar, oil, lemon juice and seasoning and mix well.

2. Add the chicken breasts and coat with the mixture generously.

3. Refrigerate to marinate for about 25-30 minutes.

4. Preheat the grill to medium heat.

5. Grease the grill grate.

6.Remove the chicken from bowl and discard the remaining marinade.

7.Place the chicken breasts onto the grill and cover with the lid.

8.Cook for about 5-7 minutes per side or until desired doneness.

9.Serve hot alongside the kale.

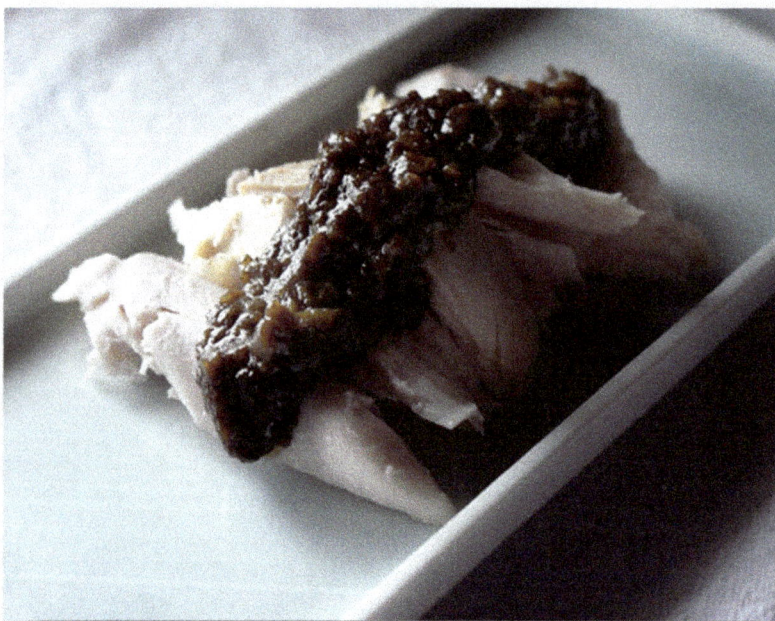

Lemony Chicken Thighs

Prep Time: 10 minutes

Cook Time: 16 minutes

Serve: 4

Ingredients:

- 2 tablespoons olive oil, divided
- 1 tablespoon fresh lemon juice
- 1 tablespoon lemon zest, grated
- 2 teaspoons dried oregano
- 1 teaspoon dried thyme
- Salt and ground black pepper, to taste
- 1½ pounds bone-in chicken thighs
- 6 cups fresh baby spinach

Instructions:

1.Preheat your oven to 420 degree F.

2.Add 1 tablespoon of the oil, lemon juice, lemon zest, dried herbs, salt, and black pepper in a big-mixing bowl and mix well.

3.Add the chicken thighs and coat with the mixture generously.

4.Refrigerate to marinate for at least 20 minutes.

5.In an oven-proof wok, heat the remaining oil over medium-high heat and sear the chicken thighs for about 2–3 minutes per side.

6.Immediately transfer the wok into the oven and Bake for approximately 10 minutes.

7.Serve hot alongside the spinach.

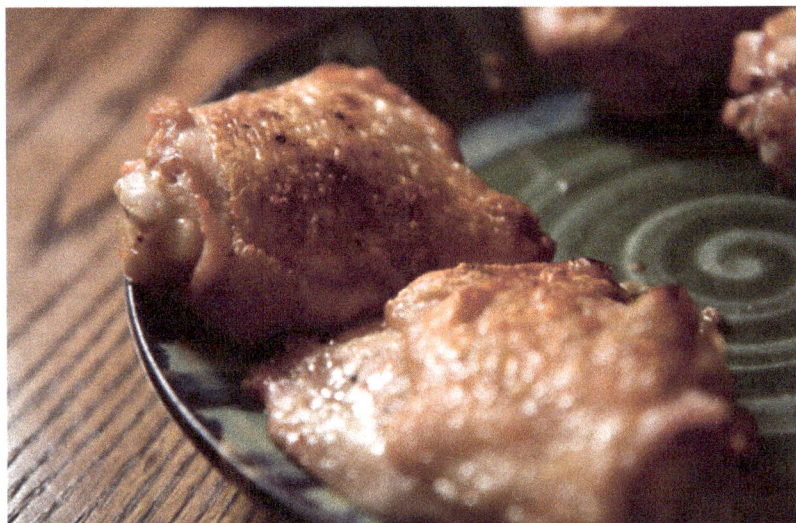

Spicy Chicken Drumsticks

Prep Time: 10 minutes

Cook Time: 40 minutes

Serve: 5

Ingredients:

- 2 tablespoons avocado oil
- 1 tablespoon fresh lime juice
- 1 teaspoon red chili powder
- 1 teaspoon garlic powder
- Salt, as required
- 5 (8-ounce) chicken drumsticks
- 8 cups fresh baby arugula

Instructions:

1.In a mixing bowl, mix avocado oil, lime juice, chili powder and garlic powder and mix well.

2.Add the chicken-drumsticks and coat with the marinade generously.

3.Cover the bowl and refrigerate for about 30-60 minutes to marinate.

4.Preheat your grill to medium-high heat.

5.Place the chicken drumsticks onto the grill and cook for about 30-40 minutes, flipping after every 5 minutes.

6.Serve hot alongside the arugula.

Baked Chicken & Bell Peppers

Prep Time: 15 minutes

Cook Time: 25 minutes

Serve: 4

Ingredients:

- 1-pound boneless, skinless chicken breasts, cut into thin strips ½ of green bell pepper, seeded and cut into strips
- ½ of red bell pepper, seeded and cut into strips 1 medium onion, sliced 2 tablespoons olive oil
- ½ teaspoon dried oregano
- 2 teaspoons chili powder
- 1½ teaspoons ground cumin
- 1 teaspoon garlic powder
- Salt, to taste

Instructions:

1. Preheat your oven to 400 degrees F.

2. In a tub, add all of the ingredients and mix well.

3. Place the chicken mixture into a 9x13-inch baking dish and spread in an even layer.

4.Bake for about 22-25 minutes, or until the chicken is completely cooked.

Tofu & Veggie Salad

Prep Time: 20 minutes

Serve: 8

Ingredients:

For Dressing:

- ¼ cup balsamic vinegar
- ¼ cup low-sodium soy sauce
- 2 tablespoons water
- 1 teaspoon sesame oil, toasted
- 1 teaspoon Sriracha
- 3-4 drops liquid stevia

For Salad:

- 1½ pounds baked firm tofu, cubed
- 2 large zucchinis, sliced thinly
- 2 large-yellow bell-peppers, seeded and sliced thinly
- 3 cups cherry tomatoes, halved
- 2 cups radishes, sliced thinly
- 2 cups purple cabbage, shredded
- 10 cups fresh baby spinach

Instructions:

1.For Dressing: in a bowl, add all the ingredients and beat until well combined.

2.Divide the chickpeas, tofu and vegetables into serving bowls.

3.Drizzle with dressing and serve immediately.

Blueberries & Spinach Salad

Prep Time: 15 minutes

Serve: 4

Ingredients:

For Salad:

- 6 cups fresh baby spinach
- 1½ cups fresh blueberries
- ¼ cup onion, sliced
- ¼ cup almond, sliced
- ¼ cup feta cheese, crumbled

For Dressing:

- 1/3 cup olive oil
- 2 tablespoons fresh lemon juice
- ¼ teaspoon liquid stevia
- 1/8 teaspoon garlic powder
- Salt, as required

Instructions:

1.For Salad: in a bowl, add the spinach, berries, onion and almonds and mix.

2.For Dressing: in another small bowl, add all the ingredients and beat until well blended.

3.Place the dressing over salad and gently toss to coat well.

Mixed Berries Salad

Prep Time: 15 minutes

 Serve: 4

Ingredients:

- 1 cup fresh strawberries, hulled and sliced ½ cups fresh blackberries
- ½ cup fresh blueberries
- ½ cup fresh raspberries
- 6 cup fresh arugula
- 2 tablespoons extra-virgin olive oil
- Salt and ground black pepper, as required

Instructions:

1.Place all the ingredients in a salad-bowl and toss to coat them well.

Kale & Citrus Fruit Salad

Prep Time: 15 minutes

Serve: 2

Ingredients:

For Salad:

- 3 cups-fresh kale, tough ribs removed and torn
- 1 orange, peeled and segmented
- 1 grapefruit, peeled and segmented
- 2 tablespoons unsweetened dried cranberries ¼ teaspoon white sesame seeds

For Dressing:

- 2 tablespoons extra-virgin olive oil
- 2 tablespoons fresh orange juice
- 1 teaspoon Dijon mustard
- ½ teaspoon raw honey
- Salt and ground black pepper, as required

Instructions:

1.For Salad: in a salad bowl, place all ingredients and mix.

2.For Dressing: place all ingredients in another bowl and beat until well combined.

3.Place dressing on top of salad and toss to coat well.

Kale, Apple & Cranberry Salad

Prep Time: 15 minutes

Serve: 4

Ingredients:

- 6 cups fresh baby kale
- 3 large apples, cored and sliced
- ¼ cup unsweetened dried cranberries
- ¼ cup almonds, sliced
- 2 tablespoons extra-virgin olive oil
- 1 tablespoon raw honey
- Salt and ground black pepper, as required

Instructions:

1.Place all the ingredients in a salad-bowl and toss to coat them well.

Rocket, Beat & Orange Salad

Prep Time: 15 minutes

Serve: 4

Ingredients:

- 3 large oranges, peeled, seeded and sectioned
- 2 beets, trimmed, peeled and sliced
- 6 cups fresh rocket
- ¼ cup walnuts, chopped
- 3 tablespoons olive oil
- Pinch of salt

Instructions:

1.In a salad bowl, place all ingredients and gently, toss to coat.

Cucumber & Tomato Salad

Prep Time: 15 minutes

Serve: 6

Ingredients:

For Salad:

- 3 large English cucumbers, sliced thinly sliced
- 2 cups tomatoes, chopped
- 6 cup lettuce, torn

For Dressing:

- 4 tablespoons olive oil
- 2 tablespoons balsamic vinegar
- 1 tablespoon fresh lemon juice
- Salt and ground black pepper, as required

Instructions:

1.For Salad: in a big-bowl, add the cucumbers, onion and dill and mix.

2.For Dressing: in a small bowl, add all the ingredients and beat until well combined.

3.Place the dressing over the salad and toss to coat well.

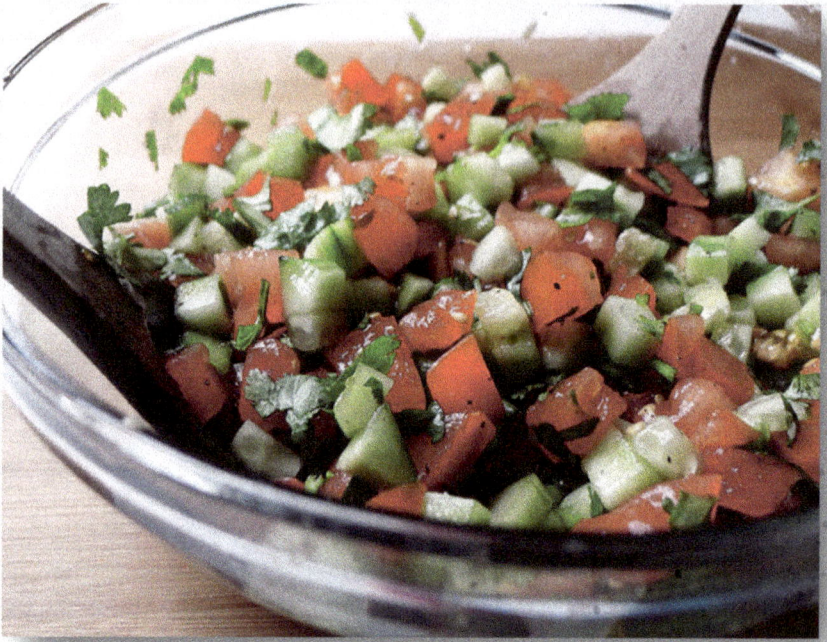

Mixed Veggie Salad

Prep Time: 20 minutes

Serve: 6

Ingredients:

For Dressing:

- 1 small avocado, peeled, pitted and chopped
- ¼ cup low-fat plain Greek yogurt
- 1 small yellow onion, chopped
- 1 garlic clove, chopped
- 2 tablespoons fresh parsley
- 2 tablespoons fresh lemon juice

For Salad:

- 6 cups fresh spinach, shredded
- 2 medium zucchinis, cut into thin slices
- ½ cup celery, sliced
- ½ cup red bell pepper, seeded and sliced thinly
- ½ cup yellow onion, sliced thinly
- ½ cup cucumber, sliced thinly
- ½ cup cherry tomatoes, halved
- ¼ cup Kalamata olives, pitted

- ½ cup feta cheese, crumbled

Instructions:

1.For Dressing: in a food processor, add all the ingredients and pulse until smooth.

2.For Salad: in a salad bowl, add all the ingredients and mix well.

3.Pour the dressing over the salad, throw it gently and cover it well.

Eggs & Veggie Salad

Prep Time: 15 minutes

Serve: 8

Ingredients:

For Salad:

- 2 large English cucumbers, sliced thinly sliced
- 2 cups tomatoes, chopped
- 8 hard-boiled eggs, peeled and sliced
- 8 cups fresh baby spinach

For Dressing:

- 4 tablespoons olive oil
- 2 tablespoons balsamic vinegar
- 1 tablespoon fresh lemon juice
- Salt and ground black pepper, as required

Instructions:

1.For Salad: in a salad bowl, add the cucumbers, onion and dill and mix.

2.For Dressing: in a small bowl, add all the ingredients and beat until well blended.

3.Place the dressing over the salad and toss to coat well.

Chicken & Orange Salad

Prep Time: 15 minutes

Cook Time: 16 minutes

Serve: 5

Ingredients:

For Chicken:

- 4 (6-ounce) boneless, skinless-chicken breast halves Salt and ground black pepper, as required 2 tablespoons extra-virgin olive oil

For Salad:

- 8 cups fresh baby arugula
- 5 medium oranges, peeled and sectioned
- 1 cup onion, sliced

For Dressing:

- 2 tablespoons extra-virgin olive oil
- 2 tablespoons fresh orange juice
- 2 tablespoons balsamic vinegar
- 1½ teaspoons shallots, minced
- 1 garlic clove, minced
- Salt and ground black pepper, as required

Instructions:

1.For chicken: season each chicken breast half with salt and black pepper evenly.

2.Place chicken over a rack set in a rimmed baking sheet.

3.Refrigerate for at least 30 minutes.

4.Remove the baking sheet from refrigerator and pat dry the chicken breast halves with paper towels.

5.Heat the oil in a 12-inch sauté pan over medium-low heat.

6.Place the chicken breast halves, smooth-side down, and cook for about 9-10 minutes, without moving.

7.Flip the chicken breasts and cook for about 6 minutes or until cooked through.

8.Remove the sauté pan from heat and let the chicken stand in the pan for about 3 minutes.

9.Transfer the chicken breasts onto a cutting board for about 5 minutes.

10.Cut each chicken breast half into desired-sized slices.

11.For Salad: place all ingredients in a salad bowl and mix.

12.Add chicken slices and stir to combine.

13.For Dressing: place all ingredients in another bowl and beat until well combined.

14.Place the salad onto each serving plate.

15.Drizzle with dressing.

Chicken & Strawberry Salad

Prep Time: 20 minutes

Cook Time: 16 minutes

Serve: 8

Ingredients:

- 2 pounds boneless, skinless chicken breasts ½ cup olive oil
- ¼ cup fresh lemon juice
- 2 tablespoons Erythritol
- 1 garlic clove, minced
- Salt and ground black pepper, as required 4 cups fresh strawberries
- 8 cups fresh spinach, torn

Instructions:

1.For marinade: in a large bowl, add oil, lemon juice, Erythritol, garlic, salt and black pepper and beat until well combined.

2.In a big-resealable plastic bag, place chicken and ¾ cup marinade.

3.Seal bag and shake to coat well.

4.Refrigerate overnight.

5.Cover the bowl of remaining marinade and refrigerate before serving.

6.Preheat the grill to medium heat. Grease the grill grate.

7.Remove the chicken from bag and discard the marinade.

8.Place the chicken onto grill grate and grill, covered for about 5-8 minutes per side.

9.Remove chicken from grill and cut into bite sized pieces.

10.In a large bowl, add the chicken pieces, strawberries and spinach and mix.

11.Place the reserved marinade and toss to coat.

Chicken & Fruit Salad

Prep Time: 15 minutes

Serve: 4

Ingredients:

For Vinaigrette:

- 2 tablespoons apple cider vinegar
- 2 tablespoons extra-virgin olive-oil
- Salt and freshly ground black-pepper, to taste
- For Salad:
- 2 cup cooked chicken, cubed
- 4 cup lettuce, torn
- 1 large apple, peeled, cored and chopped
- 1 cup fresh strawberries, hulled and sliced

Instructions:

1.For vinaigrette: in a small bowl, add all ingredients and beat well.

2.For Salad: in a big-salad bowl, mix together all ingredients.

3.Place vinaigrette over chicken mixture and toss to coat well.

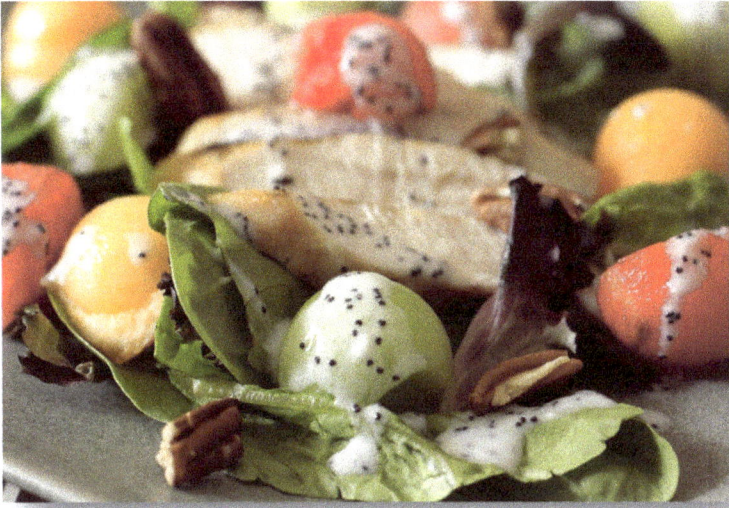

Chicken, Tomato & Arugula Salad

Prep Time: 15 minutes

Cook Time: 15 minutes

Serve: 4

Ingredients:

For Chicken:

- 3 (6-ounce) skinless, boneless chicken breast halves
- 2 teaspoons orange zest, grated finely
- 1/3 cup fresh orange juice
- 4 garlic cloves, minced
- 2 tablespoons maple syrup
- 1½ teaspoons dried thyme, crushed

For Salad:

- 6 cups fresh baby arugula
- 2 cups cherry tomatoes, quartered
- 3 tablespoons extra-virgin olive oil
- 2 tablespoons fresh lime juice
- Salt and ground black pepper, as required

Instructions:

1.For chicken: in a zip lock bag, all the ingredients.

2.Seal the bag and shake to coat well.

3.Refrigerate to marinate for about 6-8 hours, flipping occasionally.

4.Preheat the oven to broiler.

5.Line a broiler pan with a piece of foil.

6.Arrange the oven rack about 6-inch away from heating element.

7.Remove the chicken breasts from bag and discard the marinade.

8.Arrange the chicken breasts onto the prepared pan in a single layer.

9.Broil for about for 15 minutes, flipping once halfway through.

10.Remove the chicken breasts from oven and place onto a cutting board for about 10 minutes.

11.Cut the chicken breasts into desired sized slices.

12.For Salad: in a bowl, add all ingredients and toss to coat well.

13.Add chicken slices and stir to combine.

Egg on Avocado Toast

Prep Time: 3 minutes

Cook Time: 5 minutes

Serve: 1

Ingredients:

- slice bread
- salt and pepper to taste
- 1 tbsp. olive oil
- Sriracha
- 1 egg
- 1 tbsp. lemon
- ½ medium avocado

Instructions:

1.On medium-high heat, fry the egg and the toast in the pan with the olive oil.

2.In the meantime, mash the avocado, add salt and pepper, and put some lemon to the mixture.

3.Now add an egg to your toast.

4.Put a little bit of Sriracha and munches (or your favorite spicy sauce).

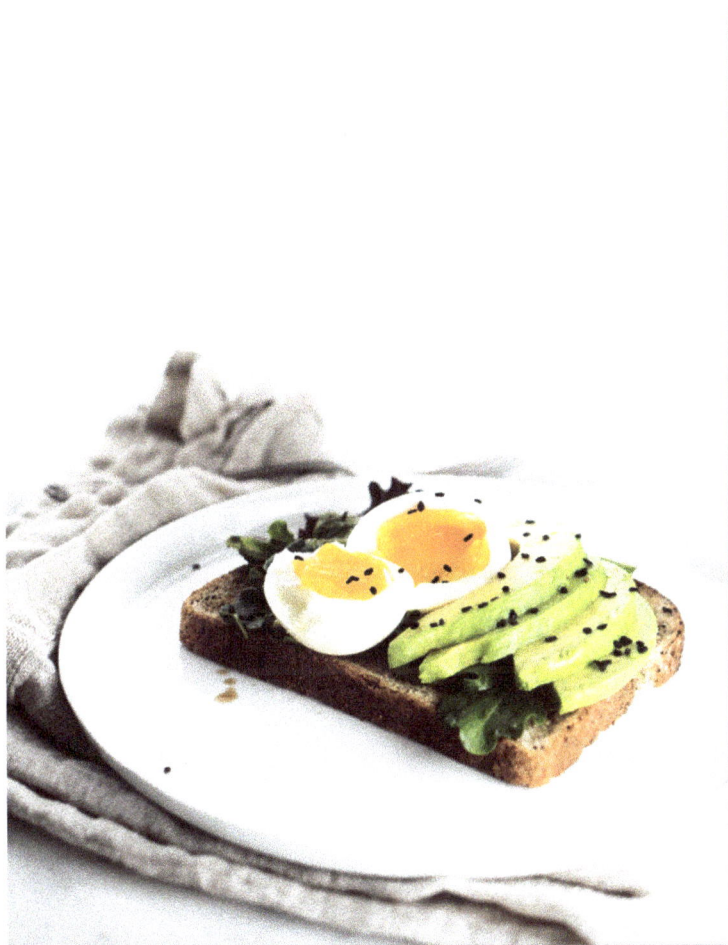

Moroccan Couscous Salad

Prep Time: 30 min

Cook Time: None

Serve: 6

Ingredients:

- 2 tbsp. olive oil
- fig, fresh (don't worry if you can't find one)
- ½ orange's zest
- orange
- 1 medium zucchini
- 1 pomegranate
- 1 tbsp. ginger powder (fresh is fine too. Chop it finely.)
- tbsp. cumin
- 1 tbsp. paprika powder
- 1 bell pepper, red
- ½ cup parsley, fresh
- 1 tbsp. salt
- salt and pepper to taste
- 1 cup of water
- ¼ cup raisins
- 1 cup instant couscous

- Optional
- bunch radish (thinly sliced)

Instructions:

1.Boil water in a wide serving bowl and apply it to the couscous.

2.Cover a tea towel or lid with the couscous and leave for 5 minutes.

3.Gently loosen the couscous with a fork and add the cumin, ginger, olive oil, and paprika powder. You want it dry and cool, no big clumps.

4.Wash the cherry, rub the zest.

5.Peel and chop the orange and, along with the zest, add it to the salad.

6.Deseed and apply the seeds to the pomegranate.

7.Finely cut the zucchini and thinly slice the red pepper. To the salad, add them.

8.Cut it upp and add it to the salad if you've managed to find a fig.

9.Clean the parsley and any other optional herbs, chop them, and then return them to the salad again.

10. Give a decent toss to it. It's that easy!

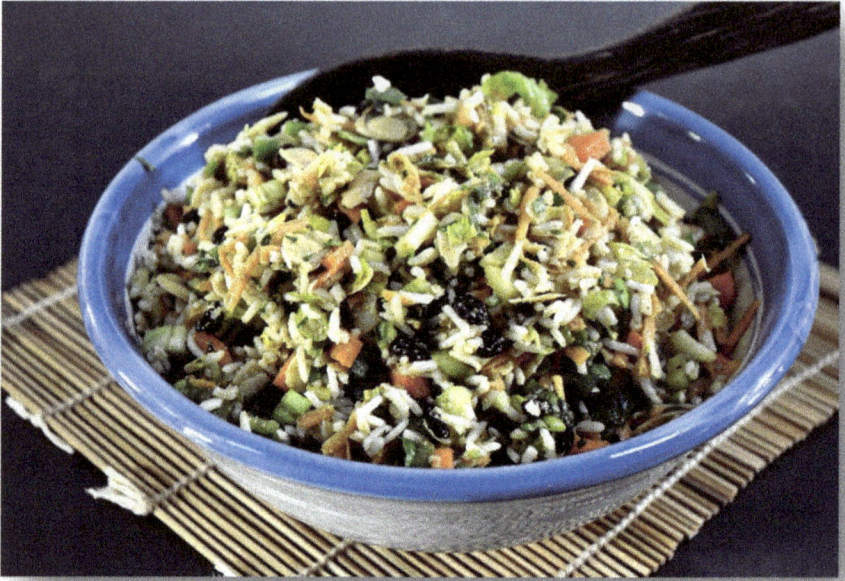

Chicken Breast with Asparagus

Prep Time: 15 minutes

Cook Time: 16 minutes

Serve: 5

Ingredients:

For Chicken:

- ¼ cup extra-virgin olive oil
- ¼ cup fresh lemon juice
- 2 tablespoons maple syrup
- 1 garlic clove, minced
- Salt and ground black pepper, as required
- 5 (6-ounce) boneless, skinless chicken breasts

For Asparagus:

- 1½ pounds fresh asparagus
- 2 tablespoons extra-virgin olive oil

Instructions:

1.For marinade: in a large bowl, add oil, lemon juice, Erythritol, garlic, salt and black pepper and beat until well combined.

2.In a large-resealable plastic-bag, place the chicken and ¾ cup of marinade.

3.Seal the bag and shake to coat well.

4.Refrigerate overnight.

5.Cover the bowl of remaining marinade and refrigerate before serving.

6.Preheat the grill to medium heat. Grease the grill grate.

7.Remove the chicken from bag and discard the marinade.

8.Place the chicken onto grill grate and grill, covered for about 5-8 minutes per side.

9.Meanwhile, in a pan of boiling water, arrange a steamer basket.

10. Place the asparagus in steamer basket and steam, covered for about 5-7 minutes.

11. Drain the asparagus well and transfer into a bowl.

12. Add oil and toss to coat well.

13. Divide the chicken breasts and asparagus onto serving plates and serve.

Chicken with Zoodles

Prep Time: 15 minutes

Cook Time: 18 minutes

Serve: 4

Ingredients:

- 2 cups zucchini, spiralized with Blade
- Salt, to taste
- 1½ pounds boneless, skinless chicken breasts Freshly ground black pepper, to taste
- 1 tablespoon olive oil
- 1 cup low-fat plain Greek yogurt
- ¼ cup low-fat Parmesan cheese, shredded ½ cup low-sodium chicken broth
- ½ teaspoon Italian seasoning
- ½ teaspoon garlic powder
- 1 cup fresh spinach, chopped
- 3-6 slices sun-dried tomatoes
- 1 tablespoon garlic, chopped

Instructions:

1.Preheat your oven to 350 degrees F.

2.Line a large-baking-sheet with a parchment paper.

3.Place the zucchini noodles and salt onto the prepared baking sheet and toss to coat well.

4.Arrange the zucchini-noodles in an even layer and Bake for approximately 15 minutes.

5.Meanwhile, season the chicken breasts with salt and black pepper.

6.In a large-skillet, heat the oil over medium-high heat and cook the chicken breasts for about 4-5 minutes per side or until cooked through.

7.With a slotted spoon, transfer the cooked chicken onto a plate and set aside.

8.In the same skillet, add the yogurt, Parmesan cheese, broth, Italian seasoning and garlic powder and beat until well combined.

9.Place the skillet over medium-high-heat and cook for about 2-3 minutes or until it starts to thicken, stirring continuously.

10.Stir in the spinach, sun-dried tomatoes and garlic and cook for about 2-3 minutes.

11. Attach the chicken breasts, then cook for 1-2 minutes or so.

12.Divide the zucchini noodles onto serving plates and top each with chicken mixture.

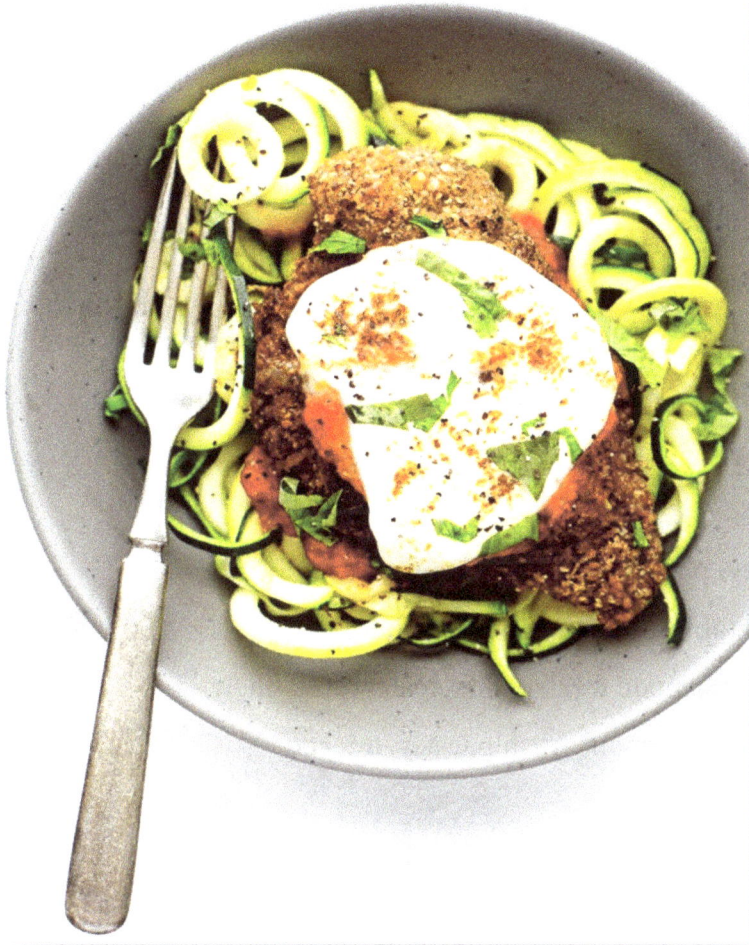

Chicken with Yellow Squash

Prep Time: 15 minutes

Cook Time: 17 minutes

Serve: 6

Ingredients:

- 2 tablespoons olive oil, divided
- 1½ pounds skinless, boneless-chicken breasts, cut into bite-sized pieces
- Salt and freshly ground black-pepper, to taste 2 garlic cloves, minced
- 1½ pounds yellow squash, sliced
- 2 tablespoons fresh lemon juice
- 1 teaspoon fresh lemon zest, grated finely
- 2 tablespoons fresh parsley, minced

Instructions:

1.Heat 1 normal spoon of oil in a large skillet over medium heat and fry the chicken for around 6-8 minutes, or until golden brown on all sides.

2.Transfer the chicken onto a plate.

3.Heat the remaining oil over medium heat in the same skillet and sauté the garlic for approximately 1 minute.

4.Add the squash slices and cook for about 5-6 minutes,

5.Stir in the chicken and cook for about 2 minutes.

6. Remove from heat and apply-lemon juice to whisk, zest and parsley.

Chicken with Bell Peppers

Prep Time: 15 minutes

Cook Time: 20 minutes

Serve: 6

Ingredients:

- 3 tablespoons olive oil, divided
- 1 yellow bell pepper, seeded and sliced
- 1 red bell pepper, seeded and sliced
- 1 green bell pepper, seeded and sliced
- 1 medium onion, sliced
- 1-pound boneless, skinless chicken breasts, sliced thinly1 teaspoon dried oregano, crushed
- ¼ teaspoon garlic powder
- ¼ teaspoon ground cumin
- Salt and freshly ground black-pepper, to taste
- ¼ cup low-sodium chicken broth

Instructions:

1.In a skillet, heat 1 normal spoon of oil over medium-high heat and cook the bell peppers and onion slices for about 4-5 minutes.

2.With a slotted spoon, transfer the peppers mixture onto a plate.

3.In the same skillet, heat the remaining oil over medium-high heat and cook the chicken for about 8 minutes, stirring frequently.

4.Stir in the thyme, spices, salt, black pepper, and broth, and bring to a boil.

5.Add the peppers mixture and stir to combine.

6. Reduce the heat to medium and cook, stirring periodically, for around 3-5 minutes or until all the liquid is absorbed.

Chicken with Mushrooms

Prep Time: 15 minutes

Cook Time: 20 minutes

Serve: 4

Ingredients:

- 2 tablespoons almond flour
- Salt and freshly ground black-pepper, to taste
- 4 (4-ounce) skinless, boneless chicken breasts
- 2 tablespoons olive oil
- 6 garlic cloves, chopped
- ¾ pound fresh mushrooms, sliced
- ¾ cup low-sodium chicken broth
- ¼ cup balsamic vinegar
- 1 bay leaf
- ¼ teaspoon dried thyme

Instructions:

1. Mix the rice, salt and black pepper together in a dish.

2.Coat the chicken breasts with flour mixture evenly.

3.In a skillet, heat the olive-oil over medium-high heat and stir fry chicken for about 3 minutes.

4.Add the garlic and flip the chicken breasts.

5.Spread mushrooms over chicken and cook for about 3 minutes, shaking the skillet frequently.

6.Add the broth, vinegar, bay leaf and thyme and stir to combine.

7. Lower the heat to medium-low, cover and simmer for about 10 minutes, occasionally tossing the chicken.

8. Move the chicken with a slotted spoon to a warm serving platter and cover it with a piece of foil to keep it warm.

9.Place the pan of sauce over medium-high heat and cook, uncovered for about 7 minutes.

10.Remove the pan from heat and discard the bay leaf.

11.Place mushroom sauce over chicken and serve hot.

Chicken with Broccoli

Prep Time: 15 minutes

Cook Time: 22 minutes

Serve: 4

Ingredients:

- 2 tablespoons olive oil, divided
- 4 (4-ounce) boneless, skinless chicken breasts, cut into small-pieces
- Salt and freshly ground black-pepper, 1 onion to taste, finely chopped
- 1 teaspoon fresh ginger, grated
- 1 teaspoon garlic, minced
- 1 cup broccoli florets
- 1½ cups fresh mushrooms, sliced
- 8 ounces low-sodium chicken broth

Instructions:

1.In a large skillet, heat 1 normal spoon of oil over medium-high heat and stir fry the chicken pieces, salt, and black pepper for about 4-5 minutes or until golden brown.

2.With a grooved spoon, transfer the chicken onto a plate.

3.In the same skillet, heat the remaining-oil over medium-high heat and sauté the onion, ginger, and garlic for about 4-5 minutes.

4.Add in mushrooms and cook for about 4-5 minutes, stirring frequently.

5.Add the broccoli and stir fry for about 3 minutes.

6.Add the cooked chicken and broth and stir fry for about 3-5 minutes

7.Add in the salt and black-pepper and remove from the heat.

Chicken & Veggies Stir Fry

Prep Time: 15 minutes

Cook Time: 15 minutes

Serve: 6

Ingredients:

- 2 tablespoons fresh lime juice
- 2 tablespoons fish sauce
- 1½ teaspoons arrowroot starch
- 4 teaspoons olive oil, divided
- 1-pound skinless, boneless chicken tenders, cubed
- 1 teaspoon fresh ginger, minced
- 2 garlic cloves, minced
- ¾ teaspoon red pepper flakes, crushed
- ¼ cup water
- 4 cups broccoli, cut into bite-sized pieces
- 3 cup red-bell-pepper, seeded and sliced
- ¼ cup pine nuts

Instructions:

1.In a bowl, add lime juice, fish sauce, and arrowroot starch and mix until well combined. Set aside.

2.In a large non-stick sauté pan, heat 2 teaspoons of oil over high heat and cook chicken about 6-8 minutes, stirring frequently.

3. Move the chicken and set it aside in a dish.

4.In the same sauté pan, heat remaining oil over medium heat and sauté ginger, garlic and red pepper flakes for about 1 minute.

5.Add water, broccoli and bell pepper and stir fry for about 2-3 minutes.

6.Stir in chicken and lime juice mixture and cook for about 2-3 minutes.

7.Stir in pine nuts and immediately remove from heat.

Chicken & Broccoli Bake

Prep Time: 15 minutes

Cook Time: 24 minutes

Serve: 6

Ingredients:

- Olive oil cooking spray
- 6 (6-ounce) skinless, boneless chicken thighs
- 3 broccoli heads, cut into florets
- 4 garlic cloves, minced
- ¼ cup extra-virgin olive oil
- 1 teaspoon dried oregano, crushed
- 1 teaspoon dried rosemary
- Salt and freshly ground black-pepper, to taste

Instructions:

1.Preheat your oven to 375 degrees F.

2.Grease a large-baking dish with cooking spray.

3.In a big-bowl, add all the ingredients and toss to coat well.

4.In the bottom of the prepared baking-dish, arrange the broccoli florets and top with chicken breasts in a single layer.

5.Bake for approximately 45 minutes.

www.ingramcontent.com/pod-product-compliance
Lightning Source LLC
Chambersburg PA
CBHW050754030426
42336CB00012B/1807